EFFECTIVE NATURAL JOINT PAIN RELIEF

Harnessing Nature's Remedies for Joint Pain Recovery

ALBERT D MONK

Copyright © 2023 by Albert D Monk

DEDICATION

This book is dedicated to all those bravely battling joint pain, May this guide to Effective Natural Joint Pain Relief bring you the comfort and relief you deserve. Your strength and resilience inspire us, and it is our hope that these solutions provide you with the freedom to move and live life to the fullest once again.

Table of Contents

INTRODUCTION

Effective natural joint pain relief is a paramount concern for those who suffer from the discomfort and limitations of joint-related issues. Joint pain, often caused by conditions like arthritis, overuse, or injury, can significantly impede one's quality of life, hindering mobility and causing chronic discomfort.

In response, many individuals seek alternatives to conventional medication and invasive treatments. Natural remedies have gained prominence as viable options for managing joint pain, offering relief without the potential side effects associated with pharmaceuticals.

The allure of natural joint pain relief lies in its holistic approach, addressing not only the symptoms but also the underlying causes of discomfort.

From herbal supplements and dietary adjustments to exercise routines and mindfulness practices, a diverse range of natural solutions are being explored.

These approaches aim to reduce inflammation, promote joint health, and improve overall well-being.

This article delves into the realm of effective natural joint pain relief, offering insights into various methods that have garnered attention in the medical community and among individuals seeking a more integrative approach to managing joint discomfort.

By understanding these alternatives, readers can make informed decisions about their health and explore options that resonate with their preferences and lifestyles.

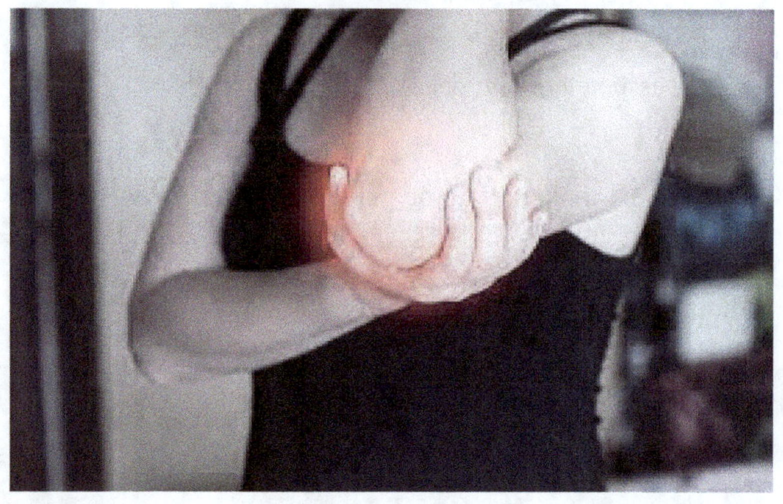

CHAPTER 1

Understanding Joint Pain

Joint pain is a widespread medical condition that affects people of all ages. It can be caused by a variety of factors, including age, injury, medical conditions, and lifestyle choices.

This chapter aims to provide a comprehensive understanding of joint pain and highlight the significance of using natural remedies to manage and alleviate this discomfort.

Joint pain, also known as arthralgia, refers to the discomfort, soreness, or inflammation experienced in the areas where two or more bones meet. Joints serve as the connectors between bones, allowing movement and flexibility.

However, when these joints are compromised, they can lead to pain and restricted mobility. Common types of joint pain include osteoarthritis, rheumatoid arthritis, gout, and injuries.

Causes of Joint Pain

1. Age: As people grow older, the wear and tear on joints increase, often resulting in conditions like osteoarthritis.

2. Injuries: Trauma from accidents, sports, or repetitive strain can damage joints, leading to pain and discomfort.

3. Medical Conditions: Conditions such as rheumatoid arthritis, lupus, and fibromyalgia can cause chronic joint pain.

4. Inflammation: Inflammation around the joints can be due to various factors, including autoimmune responses and infections.

5. Lifestyle Factors: Obesity, lack of physical activity, and poor posture can contribute to joint pain by putting extra stress on the joints.

Importance of Natural Remedies

In recent years, there has been a growing interest in natural remedies for managing joint pain. Natural remedies are often preferred due to their potential to alleviate pain and discomfort without the side effects commonly associated with pharmaceutical medications.

Some key reasons for the importance of natural remedies include:

1. Reduced Side Effects: Unlike pharmaceutical drugs, many natural remedies have minimal to no side effects, making them a safer choice for long-term use.

2. Holistic Approach: Natural remedies often focus on overall health and wellness, addressing the root causes of joint pain rather than just the symptoms.

3. Anti-Inflammatory Properties: Certain herbs and supplements possess anti-inflammatory properties that can help reduce joint inflammation and pain.

4. Nutritional Support: Natural remedies can provide essential nutrients that support joint health, such as omega-3 fatty acids, antioxidants, and vitamins.

5. Improved Mobility: Exercises like yoga, tai chi, and gentle stretching can enhance joint flexibility and mobility, reducing pain and stiffness.

6. Psychological Benefits: Natural remedies often include practices like meditation and mindfulness, which can help manage stress and contribute to pain reduction.

7. Personalized Approach: Natural remedies can be tailored to individual needs, considering factors such as diet, lifestyle, and underlying health conditions.

Common Natural Remedies for Joint Pain

1. Turmeric: Contains curcumin, which has potent anti-inflammatory effects.
Ginger: Possesses anti-inflammatory and analgesic properties.

2. Omega-3 Fatty Acids: Found in fish oil, these fats can help reduce inflammation.

3. Glucosamine and Chondroitin: Supplements that support cartilage health and reduce pain.

4. Epsom Salt Baths: Can soothe joint pain and relax muscles.

5. Acupuncture: Traditional practice involving inserting needles into specific points to alleviate pain.

6. Heat and Cold Therapy: Applying heat or cold can help relieve pain and reduce inflammation.

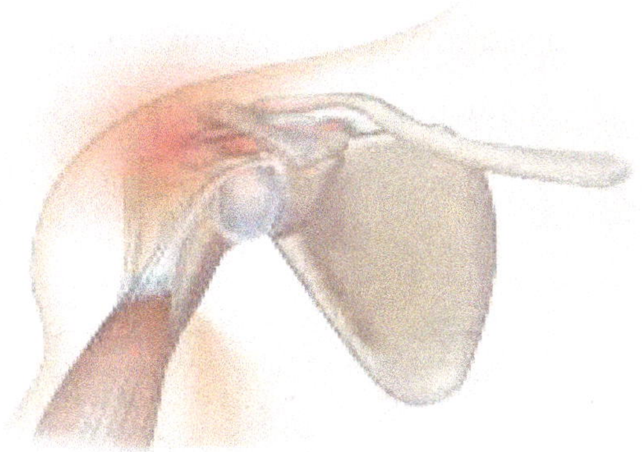

CHAPTER 2

Anatomy of Joints

Joints, also known as articulations, are the points where two or more bones meet, allowing for movement and functional interaction within the skeletal system. The anatomy of joints is crucial to understanding their structure and function. There are various types of joints in the human body, each with its unique characteristics and mobility capabilities.

Structure of Joints

Types of Joints:

Joints can be categorized into three main types based on their structure and function: fibrous joints, cartilaginous joints, and synovial joints.

1. Fibrous Joints: Fibrous joints are characterized by the presence of fibrous connective tissue between bones. These joints allow minimal movement and provide stability.

Examples of fibrous joints include sutures in the skull and syndesmoses in the forearm and lower leg.

2. Cartilaginous Joints: Cartilaginous joints are connected by cartilage, a firm but flexible connective tissue. These joints offer limited movement and are primarily designed for shock absorption. Two subtypes of cartilaginous joints exist: synchondroses and symphyses.

- Synchondroses, found in growth plates of developing bones, are connected by hyaline cartilage.

- Symphyses, such as the intervertebral discs and pubic symphysis, are united by fibrocartilage and provide a degree of flexibility while maintaining stability.

3. Synovial Joints: Synovial joints are the most versatile and abundant type of joints in the body. These joints possess a synovial cavity, which is filled with synovial fluid, allowing for smooth movement between articulating bones. Synovial joints are further classified based on their shape and movement potential:

- Articular Cartilage: Smooth and slippery cartilage that covers the ends of bones, reducing friction and allowing smooth movement.

- Synovial Cavity: A space between the articulating bones filled with synovial fluid, which lubricates and nourishes the joint.

- Synovial Membrane: Lines the joint capsule and produces synovial fluid.

- Joint Capsule: Surrounds the joint, consisting of an outer fibrous layer and an inner synovial membrane.

- Ligaments: Connect bones and help stabilize the joint.

- Bursae: Small fluid-filled sacs that reduce friction between tendons, ligaments, and bones.

- Menisci: Crescent-shaped cartilages in certain joints (e.g., knee) that provide cushioning and stability.

Functions of Joints

1. Movement: Joints facilitate a wide range of movements, including flexion (bending), extension (straightening), abduction (moving away from the body's midline), adduction (moving toward the body's midline), rotation, and circumduction (circular motion).

2. Support: Joints provide structural support to the body, allowing it to maintain an upright posture against gravity.

3. Protection: Some joints, like those in the skull, protect vital organs like the brain.

4. Shock Absorption: Cartilaginous joints, synovial fluid, and menisci help absorb and distribute forces during movement, reducing impact on bones.

5. Synovial Fluid Production: Synovial joints produce synovial fluid that lubricates the joint surfaces, reducing friction and wear.

6. Muscle Attachment: Joints serve as attachment points for muscles and tendons, allowing movement when muscles contract.

7. Sensation: Some joints have sensory receptors called proprioceptors that provide feedback about the joint's position, aiding in balance and coordination.

Joints come in various forms and serve essential functions in the body, allowing movement, providing support, and protecting vital structures.

The diversity in joint types enables the body to perform an array of movements, from the subtlest to the most complex. Understanding the structure and function of joints is crucial for comprehending human anatomy and the mechanics of movement.

Common Joint Issues

Various factors can lead to joint issues, causing discomfort and limitations in daily activities. Some common joint issues include;

1. Osteoarthritis: This is the most prevalent joint disorder, often associated with aging. It occurs due to the progressive degeneration of the protective cartilage that cushions the ends of bones. This can lead to pain, stiffness, and reduced joint flexibility, most commonly affecting the knees, hips, and hands.

2. Rheumatoid Arthritis: An autoimmune disorder where the body's immune system mistakenly attacks the synovium, a membrane that lines the joints. This leads to inflammation, joint pain, swelling, and in severe cases, joint deformity. It can affect multiple joints symmetrically.

3. Gout: Caused by an accumulation of uric acid crystals in the joints, gout often targets the big toe. It leads to sudden, severe pain, redness, and swelling. Dietary choices, genetics, and certain health conditions can contribute to gout.

4. Bursitis: Bursae are small, fluid-filled sacs that cushion joints. When they become inflamed due to repetitive motions or pressure, it leads to bursitis. This condition causes pain and limited joint movement, particularly in the shoulders, elbows, and hips.

5. Tendinitis: Tendons connect muscles to bones, and when they become inflamed due to overuse or injury, it's known as tendinitis. It causes pain and tenderness, often near joints like the shoulders, elbows, and knees.

6. Ligament Injuries: Ligaments connect bone to bone and provide stability to joints. Injuries such as sprains and tears can occur due to sudden movements or accidents. Common examples include anterior cruciate ligament (ACL) tears in the knee.

7. Frozen Shoulder: Also known as adhesive capsulitis, this condition causes the shoulder joint to become stiff and painful, limiting its range of motion. The exact cause is often unclear, but it can result from injury, overuse, or certain medical conditions.

8. Carpal Tunnel Syndrome: Affecting the wrist joint, carpal tunnel syndrome occurs when the median nerve, which runs through the wrist, becomes compressed. This leads to numbness, tingling, and weakness in the hand.

9. Ankylosing Spondylitis: This is a type of inflammatory arthritis that primarily affects the spine. Over time, it can lead to fusion of the spinal vertebrae, causing stiffness and reduced flexibility. It can also affect other joints and lead to fatigue.

10. Joint Infections: Joints can be affected by bacterial, viral, or fungal infections. These infections can cause severe pain, swelling, redness, and fever. To avoid additional difficulties, prompt medical attention is essential.

Prevention and Management

- Keep a healthy weight to lessen strain on your joints.

- Stay physically active to strengthen muscles and support joint function.

- Practice proper ergonomics to avoid repetitive strain on joints.

- Protect joints during physical activities with appropriate gear.

- Consume a healthy, anti-inflammatory-rich diet.

- If you have a family history of joint issues, consider regular check-ups.

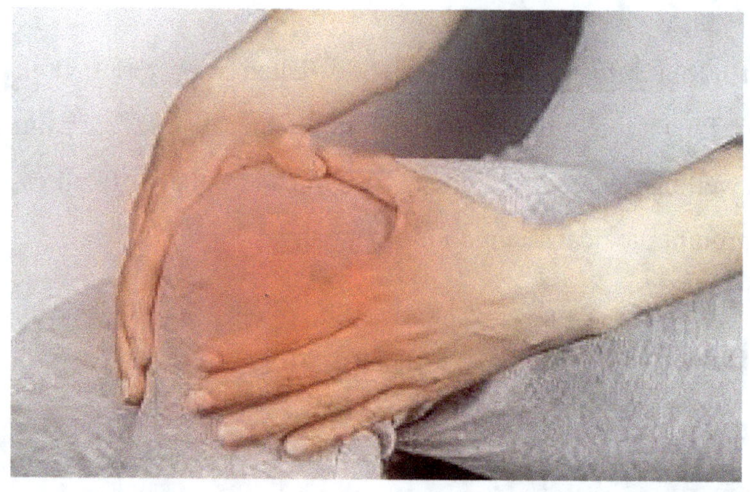

CHAPTER 3

Lifestyle Changes for Joint Health

Joint health is crucial for maintaining an active and pain-free life. Making certain lifestyle changes can significantly contribute to improving joint health and preventing conditions like arthritis. Consider the following significant factors:

Maintaining a Balanced Diet

A well-balanced diet rich in essential nutrients plays a vital role in promoting joint health. Incorporating foods rich in antioxidants, omega-3 fatty acids, and vitamins like C and D can help reduce inflammation and support the health of joints.

Foods such as fatty fish, leafy greens, nuts, and berries can provide these nutrients.

1. Staying Hydrated

Proper hydration is essential for maintaining the health of cartilage, which acts as a cushion for the joints. Drinking an adequate amount of water helps keep joints lubricated and prevents stiffness. Herbal teas and low-sugar beverages can also help you stay hydrated.

2. Regular Exercise and Physical Activity

Engaging in regular exercise is one of the most effective ways to improve joint health. Low-impact exercises like swimming, cycling, and walking help strengthen muscles around the joints, enhance flexibility, and reduce the risk of injury. It is important to establish a balance between remaining active and avoiding overexertion.

3. Importance of Proper Posture

Maintaining proper posture while sitting, standing, and performing daily activities is essential for preventing strain on joints.

Poor posture can lead to imbalances in muscle strength and contribute to joint pain. Ergonomic adjustments in workspaces and regular breaks during prolonged sitting can help maintain good posture.

4. Weight Management

Maintaining a healthy weight is crucial for joint health, particularly for weight-bearing joints like the knees and hips. Excess weight places additional stress on these joints, increasing the risk of conditions like osteoarthritis. A combination of a balanced diet and regular exercise can aid in weight management.

Incorporating these lifestyle changes can have a positive impact on joint health and overall well-being. It's important to consult with a healthcare professional before making significant changes to your lifestyle, especially if you have existing medical conditions. By taking proactive steps, you can enjoy better joint health and a higher quality of life.

CHAPTER 4

Herbal Remedies and Supplements

Joint pain is a common ailment affecting people of all ages, often attributed to conditions like arthritis, inflammation, and wear and tear. In addition to traditional medical treatments, many individuals seek relief through herbal remedies and supplements. Here are some notable options:

1. Turmeric and Curcumin: Turmeric, a vibrant yellow spice, contains an active compound called curcumin. Curcumin has potent anti-inflammatory and antioxidant properties that may help reduce joint pain.

It is believed to inhibit enzymes responsible for inflammation and play a role in managing conditions like osteoarthritis and rheumatoid arthritis.

2. Ginger: Ginger is another spice with anti-inflammatory properties. Its active components, gingerol and shogaol, have been studied for their potential to alleviate joint pain

and reduce inflammation. Ginger supplements or including fresh ginger in your diet may contribute to joint pain relief.

3. Boswellia: Also known as Indian frankincense, boswellia contains compounds that have anti-inflammatory effects. It is believed to inhibit the production of leukotrienes, which contribute to inflammation in the body.

Boswellia supplements may help manage joint pain and improve mobility, particularly in cases of osteoarthritis.

4. Omega-3 Fatty Acids: Found in fatty fish like salmon, mackerel, and sardines, omega-3 fatty acids have anti-inflammatory properties that can be beneficial for joint health.

They help balance the body's inflammatory responses and may provide relief for conditions like rheumatoid arthritis. Supplements containing omega-3 fatty acids are also available for persons who do not consume enough seafood.

5. Glucosamine and Chondroitin: Glucosamine and chondroitin are naturally occurring substances found in joint cartilage. These supplements are frequently used to treat the symptoms of osteoarthritis.

Glucosamine may support the repair of damaged cartilage, while chondroitin may help retain water and nutrients in cartilage, promoting its elasticity and shock-absorbing properties.

It's important to note that while herbal remedies and supplements may offer relief for some individuals, their efficacy can vary. Results might take time and vary depending on the underlying cause of joint pain.

Before incorporating any new supplement into your routine, it's recommended to consult a healthcare professional, especially if you're already taking medications or have existing health conditions.

Additionally, these remedies should not replace standard medical treatments, but rather complement them.

A balanced approach involving a healthy diet, regular exercise, and consultation with healthcare providers is essential for managing joint pain effectively.

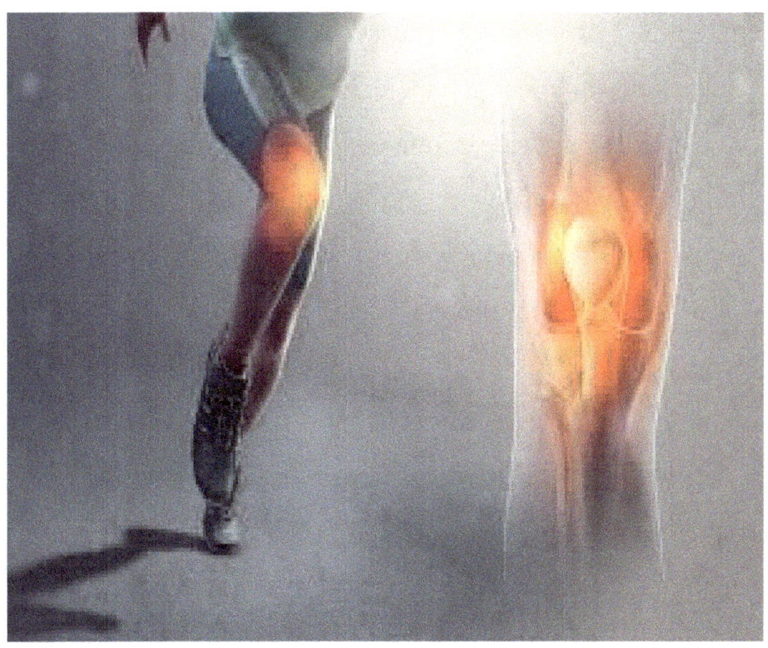

CHAPTER 5

Essential Oils for Joint Pain

Essential oils have been used for centuries to alleviate various health concerns, including joint pain. They contain concentrated plant compounds that possess anti-inflammatory, analgesic, and soothing properties. Here's a comprehensive overview of four essential oils commonly used for joint pain relief:

Lavender Oil

Lavender oil is renowned for its calming aroma and therapeutic benefits. While it's more often associated with relaxation and stress relief, it also offers benefits for joint pain.

Lavender oil's anti-inflammatory properties can help reduce swelling and discomfort around the joints. Its gentle nature makes it suitable for sensitive skin and mild pain. Massage the affected area with a mixture of a few drops of lavender oil and a carrier oil (such as coconut or almond oil) for comfort.

Eucalyptus Oil

Eucalyptus oil is well-known for its cooling and analgesic properties. Its main active compound, eucalyptol, has been studied for its anti-inflammatory effects. Eucalyptus oil can provide a soothing sensation and may help ease joint pain.

Mixing a few drops of eucalyptus oil with a carrier oil and massaging it into the affected joints might offer relief. Additionally, inhaling the vapors of eucalyptus oil through steam inhalation or a diffuser can provide a refreshing and pain-relieving experience.

Peppermint Oil

Peppermint oil contains menthol, a compound known for its cooling and pain-relieving effects. When applied topically, it can provide a numbing sensation that temporarily alleviates joint pain.

Peppermint oil also has mild anti-inflammatory properties. Mixing a few drops of peppermint oil with a carrier oil and gently massaging it onto the affected area can provide a cooling relief sensation. However, as peppermint oil is potent, it's important to dilute it properly to avoid skin irritation.

Frankincense Oil

Frankincense oil has been used for centuries in traditional medicine for its anti-inflammatory and analgesic properties. It's believed to help improve circulation, reduce swelling, and promote joint health.

Applying diluted frankincense oil topically can offer relief from joint discomfort. Its warming effect can help relax muscles and improve mobility around the joints. Mix a few drops of frankincense oil with a carrier oil and massage it onto the affected area.

It's important to note that while essential oils can provide relief, they are not a substitute for medical treatment.

If you have chronic or severe joint pain, consult a healthcare professional before using essential oils. Before using any essential oil, always conduct a patch test to be sure you won't experience an allergic response.

Additionally, pregnant women, individuals with certain medical conditions, or those taking specific medications should exercise caution and seek medical advice before using essential oils.

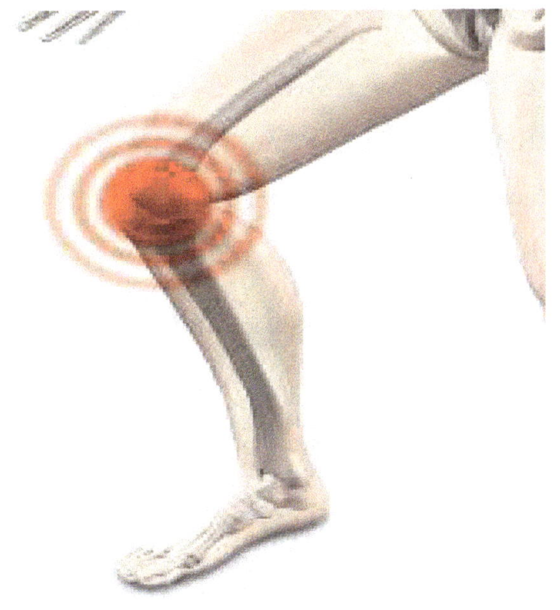

CHAPTER 6

Heat and Cold Therapy

Heat and cold therapy are common non-invasive methods used to manage pain, reduce inflammation, and promote healing. These therapies utilize the physiological effects of temperature changes to provide relief from various conditions.

Heat therapy involves applying warmth to the body, while cold therapy involves the application of cold temperatures. Both methods can be applied using heat packs and cold compresses, respectively.

Application of Heat Packs

The use of heat, commonly referred to as thermotherapy, is used to promote blood flow, relax the muscles, and reduce discomfort. Heat packs are commonly used to administer this therapy. They can be categorized into dry heat packs and moist heat packs.

1. Dry Heat Packs: These are heat packs that don't require water. Examples include electric heating pads, heat wraps, and heated gel packs. They provide a steady and controlled heat source, making them suitable for localized pain relief, muscle relaxation, and reducing stiffness.

2. Moist Heat Packs: Moist heat packs, such as warm damp towels, warm baths, and moist heating pads, utilize the combination of heat and moisture to penetrate deeper into tissues. They are often used to ease more chronic conditions like arthritis and promote healing in deeper tissues.

Application of Cold Compresses

Cold treatment, commonly known as cryotherapy, is the use of cold temperatures to limit blood flow, numb pain, and reduce inflammation. Cold compresses, which are usually ice packs or cold gel packs, are commonly used to administer cold therapy.

1. Ice Packs: Ice packs are a popular form of cold therapy. They are typically made by placing ice cubes or gel packs in

a protective covering. Ice packs work by constricting blood vessels, which reduces blood flow to the area, thereby diminishing inflammation and numbing the sensation of pain. They are particularly effective in treating acute injuries, such as sprains, strains, and bruises.

Application Considerations

When using heat and cold therapy, it's essential to consider a few factors:

1. Duration: Heat therapy is typically applied for 15-20 minutes, while cold therapy is often applied for 10-20 minutes. Longer periods of time can cause skin damage.

2. Frequency: Both therapies can be applied several times a day, but there should be a gap of at least an hour between applications to prevent tissue damage.

3. Precautions: Individuals with certain medical conditions, such as diabetes, circulatory issues, or sensory deficits,

should consult a healthcare professional before using heat or cold therapy.

4. Alternation: Some conditions might benefit from alternating between heat and cold therapy. This can help in reducing inflammation and promoting circulation.

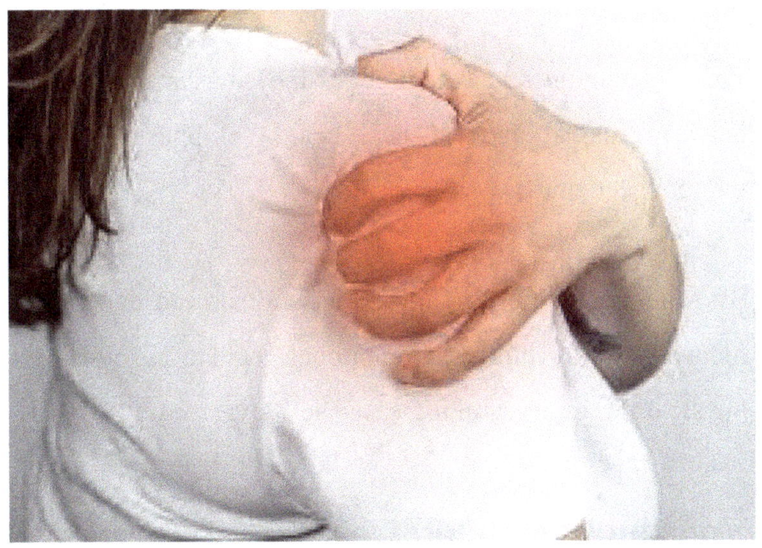

CHAPTER 7

Mind-Body Techniques

Mind-body techniques are a diverse range of practices that aim to cultivate a connection between the mind and the body, promoting holistic well-being.

These techniques acknowledge the intricate interplay between mental and physical health, emphasizing their interconnectedness.

By engaging in these practices, individuals can experience reduced stress, improved emotional regulation, enhanced physical flexibility, and increased self-awareness.

Yoga and Stretching

Yoga is a centuries-old practice that combines physical postures, breath control, meditation, and ethical principles to achieve a harmonious balance between the mind and body.

It involves a series of postures and stretches that help improve flexibility, strength, and posture. The deliberate focus on breath during yoga fosters mindfulness and stress reduction. Regular practice can lead to increased body awareness and a sense of calm.

Tai Chi

Tai Chi is a Chinese martial art that has evolved into a popular mind-body practice. It emphasizes slow, flowing movements and deep breathing to promote relaxation, balance, and mental clarity.

Practitioners move through a series of choreographed sequences, enhancing physical coordination and cultivating mindfulness. Tai Chi is frequently referred to as "meditation in motion" because of its meditative aspect.

Meditation and Deep Breathing

Meditation involves training the mind to achieve a state of heightened awareness and concentration.

It encourages the cultivation of mindfulness, leading to reduced stress and improved emotional well-being. Deep breathing techniques, often incorporated into meditation practices, activate the body's relaxation response, promoting a sense of calm and balance.

Regular meditation practice is associated with increased emotional resilience and improved focus.

Benefits of Mind-Body Techniques

1. Stress Reduction: These techniques help individuals manage and reduce stress by promoting relaxation and mindfulness, leading to a calmer state of mind.

2. Physical Well-being: Yoga, stretching, and Tai Chi enhance physical flexibility, strength, and balance, contributing to overall physical health.

3. Emotional Regulation: Meditation and deep breathing techniques empower individuals to regulate their emotions and respond to stressors more effectively.

4. Enhanced Self-Awareness: Mind-body techniques encourage self-reflection, fostering a deeper understanding of one's thoughts, feelings, and behaviors.

5. Improved Mental Focus: Regular practice can enhance concentration and cognitive function, promoting a clearer and more focused mind.

6. Holistic Wellness: By connecting the mind and body, these techniques contribute to holistic well-being, addressing both mental and physical health.

Incorporating Mind-Body Techniques

Incorporating mind-body techniques into one's routine can be highly beneficial. Begin with short sessions and gradually increase the duration as comfort and familiarity grow.

Finding a practice that resonates with you is crucial. Whether it's yoga for flexibility, Tai Chi for balance, meditation for mental clarity, or deep breathing for relaxation, consistent engagement can lead to transformative results.

CHAPTER 8

Acupuncture and Acupressure

Acupuncture and acupressure are traditional healing techniques that have been used for centuries to manage various health issues, including joint pain.

Both methods are based on the concept of stimulating specific points on the body to balance the flow of energy (often referred to as "qi" or "chi") and promote overall well-being.

These techniques have gained popularity as complementary and alternative therapies for managing joint pain and improving joint health.

Acupuncture

Acupuncture involves inserting thin needles into specific points along the body's meridians. These needles are manipulated to stimulate the flow of Qi and promote the body's natural healing response. When used to address joint pain, the needles are often placed near the affected joint or on related meridians.

Research suggests that acupuncture may help release endorphins, which are natural pain-relieving chemicals, and also influence nerve signaling to reduce pain perception.

Acupressure

Acupressure is a non-invasive technique that involves applying pressure to specific acupuncture points using fingers, thumbs, or other devices.

By pressing these points, practitioners aim to stimulate the flow of Qi and release tension in the muscles and surrounding tissues. Acupressure can be performed by a practitioner or even self-administered by the individual experiencing joint pain.

Principles and Benefits

Principles:

1. Meridian System: Both techniques are grounded in the belief that energy flows along specific meridians. These meridians correspond to various organs and body parts, including joints. By stimulating the relevant points, practitioners aim to restore balance and alleviate pain.

2. Qi Disruption: Joint pain is often seen as a result of Qi disruption or stagnation. Acupuncture and acupressure aim to restore the proper flow of Qi to relieve pain and improve overall well-being.

3. Holistic Approach: Traditional Chinese medicine takes a holistic view of the body, considering physical, emotional, and energetic aspects. Acupuncture and acupressure not only address the physical pain but also consider the underlying imbalances that may contribute to the pain.

Benefits:

Both acupuncture and acupressure have shown promising results in managing joint pain through various mechanisms:

1. Pain Relief: Stimulation of acupuncture points is thought to trigger the release of endorphins and other neurotransmitters that help reduce pain perception.

2. Inflammation Reduction: Acupuncture and acupressure may help modulate the body's inflammatory responses, potentially leading to a reduction in joint inflammation.

3. Improved Blood Flow: By promoting blood circulation around the joints, these techniques can support the delivery of oxygen and nutrients, aiding in the repair and healing process.

4. Relaxation and Stress Reduction: Both techniques induce a relaxation response, which can help alleviate muscle tension, stress, and anxiety that often exacerbate joint pain.

Effective Pressure Points

Several pressure points are commonly targeted for joint pain relief:

1. Large Intestine 4 (LI4): Located between the thumb and index finger, stimulating LI4 is believed to alleviate pain and reduce inflammation.

2. Gallbladder 34 (GB34): Found on the outer side of the leg, just below the knee, GB34 is associated with easing knee pain and promoting joint flexibility.

3. Liver 3 (LV3): Situated on the top of the foot, between the big toe and the second toe, LV3 is believed to help with general pain relief and relaxation.

4. Stomach 36 (ST36): This point is on the lower leg, below the knee. ST36 is thought to improve digestion, boost energy, and alleviate pain throughout the body.

5. Spleen 6 (SP6): Located on the inner side of the lower leg, SP6 is often targeted for various pain conditions, including joint pain and menstrual cramps.

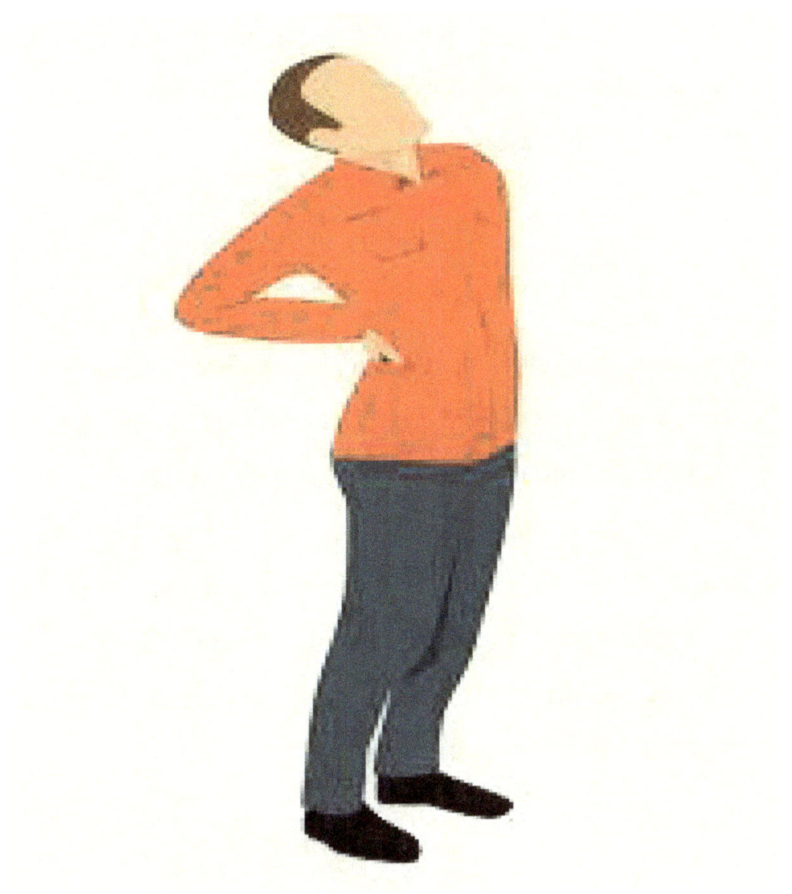

CHAPTER 9

Topical Applications

Topical applications provide a convenient and non-invasive way to manage joint discomfort. Two such options are Arnica Gel and Capsaicin Cream.

Arnica Gel

Arnica, a flowering plant from the sunflower family, has been used for centuries in traditional medicine for its potential anti-inflammatory and pain-relieving properties.

Arnica gel, derived from the arnica plant, is a popular choice for topical application to alleviate joint pain. It is available over-the-counter and is typically used for conditions such as osteoarthritis, sprains, and bruises.

Benefits:

1. Anti-Inflammatory: Arnica gel is believed to contain compounds that can help reduce inflammation, which is a common cause of joint pain.

2. Analgesic Effects: The gel is thought to have analgesic (pain-relieving) properties, providing temporary relief from mild joint discomfort.

3. Bruise and Swelling Reduction: Arnica gel is often used to minimize bruising and swelling associated with joint injuries.

Usage Precautions:

- Arnica gel should not be applied to broken or damaged skin, as it may cause irritation.

- Some people may be allergic to arnica. A patch test on a small area of skin is advisable before widespread application.

It's important to follow the recommended dosage and frequency of application, as excessive use might lead to adverse effects.

Capsaicin Cream

Capsaicin is a compound found in chili peppers, and its cream form is used topically to relieve joint pain. It works by temporarily desensitizing nerves in the area, which can reduce the perception of pain.

Benefits:

1. Nerve Desensitization: Capsaicin cream inhibits the release of a neurotransmitter called substance P, which is involved in transmitting pain signals. This desensitizes nerves, leading to reduced pain perception.

2. Long-Lasting Relief: Although the initial application might cause a burning sensation, continued use can provide prolonged relief from joint pain.

3. Non-Opioid Option: Capsaicin cream offers an alternative to oral pain medications, potentially minimizing the risks associated with opioids.

Usage Precautions:

- The initial application of capsaicin cream may cause a burning sensation. This usually diminishes with repeated use.

- Hands should be thoroughly washed after applying capsaicin cream to prevent accidentally transferring it to sensitive areas, such as the eyes.

- Capsaicin cream should be used as directed to avoid excessive irritation or adverse effects.

Topical applications like Arnica Gel and Capsaicin Cream provide unique ways to manage joint pain without relying solely on oral medications. These products offer localized relief, and their mechanisms of action complement traditional treatments.

CHAPTER 10

Dietary Considerations

Diet plays a crucial role in managing joint pain and promoting joint health. The right dietary choices can help reduce inflammation, provide essential nutrients, and support overall joint function. Here are some key considerations:

1. Anti-inflammatory Foods: Focus on consuming foods rich in antioxidants and omega-3 fatty acids. These include fruits (berries, cherries, oranges), vegetables (spinach, kale, broccoli), fatty fish (salmon, mackerel), nuts (walnuts, almonds), and seeds (flaxseeds, chia seeds).

2. Vitamins and Minerals: Adequate intake of vitamins like C, D, and E, as well as minerals like calcium, magnesium, and zinc, supports bone health. Vitamin D helps in calcium absorption, while vitamin C is essential for collagen synthesis.

3. Hydration: Staying hydrated is crucial for joint health. Water helps in maintaining lubrication and cushioning of joints. Herbal teas and low-sugar beverages can also help you stay hydrated.

4. Protein: Lean protein sources (chicken, turkey, beans, and lentils) provide amino acids necessary for tissue repair and muscle maintenance, which indirectly support joint health.

5. Whole Grains: Opt for whole grains (brown rice, quinoa, whole wheat) over refined grains. Whole grains contain fiber and nutrients that may help manage weight, reducing stress on joints.

Foods that Promote Joint Health

1. Fatty Fish: Salmon, mackerel, and sardines are rich in omega-3 fatty acids, which have anti-inflammatory properties and may help reduce joint pain.

2. Berries: Blueberries, strawberries, and cherries are packed with antioxidants that may help combat inflammation and oxidative stress.

3. Leafy Greens: Spinach, kale, and other leafy greens are high in vitamins, minerals, and antioxidants that contribute to overall joint health.

4. Nuts and Seeds: Walnuts, almonds, flaxseeds, and chia seeds provide healthy fats and essential nutrients that support joint function.

5. Oranges and Citrus: These fruits are rich in vitamin C, which is vital for collagen production and cartilage health.

6. Turmeric: The active compound in turmeric, curcumin, has anti-inflammatory effects that may alleviate joint pain.

Foods to Avoid

1. Processed Foods: Highly processed foods often contain unhealthy fats, excessive sugar, and additives that can

contribute to inflammation and weight gain, worsening joint pain.

2. Sugary Snacks and Sodas: High sugar intake can lead to weight gain and inflammation, potentially aggravating joint discomfort.

3. Red and Processed Meat: These meats can contain saturated fats that may contribute to inflammation. Limit their consumption and opt for lean protein sources.

4. Refined Grains: White bread, pasta, and other refined grains lack nutrients and fiber. They may also contribute to weight gain and inflammation.

5. Excessive Alcohol: Heavy alcohol consumption can lead to inflammation and potentially affect nutrient absorption, which could impact joint health.

6. High-Sodium Foods: Excess sodium can contribute to water retention and may worsen inflammation in some individuals.

Remember, individual responses to foods can vary. Consulting with a healthcare professional or a registered dietitian before making significant dietary changes is recommended, especially if you have specific dietary restrictions or medical conditions.

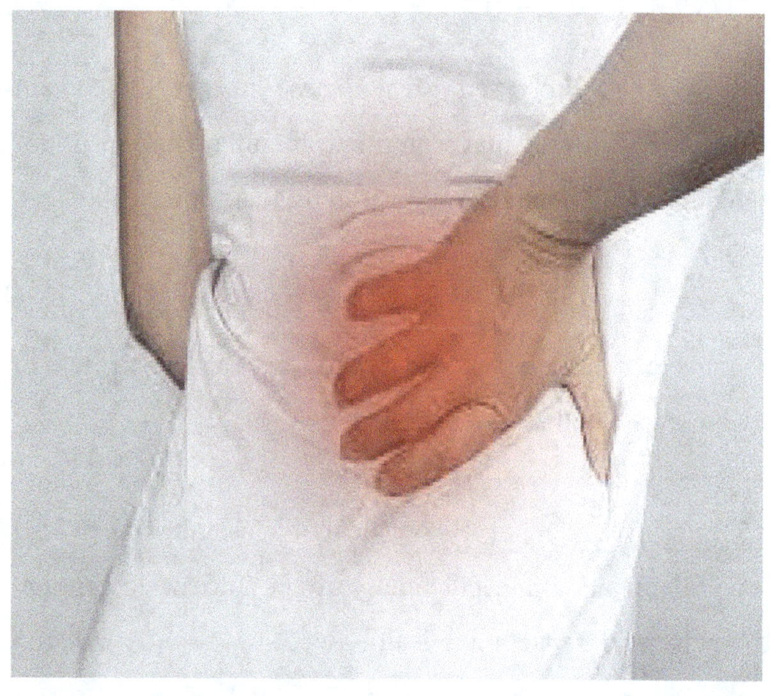

CHAPTER 11

Hydration and Joint Health

Hydration plays a crucial role in maintaining joint health and overall well-being. Joints are cushioned by synovial fluid, a lubricating substance that allows smooth movement and reduces friction between bones.

Proper hydration ensures an adequate supply of synovial fluid, helping to keep joints lubricated and functioning optimally. Inadequate hydration can lead to reduced synovial fluid production, potentially causing joint stiffness, discomfort, and even long-term joint problems.

Importance of Water Intake

Adequate water intake is essential for maintaining joint health for several reasons:

1. Synovial Fluid Production: Hydration supports the production of synovial fluid, which is essential for

lubricating and cushioning joints. Sufficient water intake helps maintain the right viscosity and volume of synovial fluid.

2. Nutrient Transport: Water carries nutrients to cells and helps remove waste products. In joints, this nutrient transport is vital for repairing tissues and maintaining joint function.

3. Shock Absorption: Joints endure impact and pressure during movement. Well-hydrated cartilage, a connective tissue that cushions joints, can better absorb shock and prevent wear and tear.

4. Inflammation Reduction: Dehydration can trigger inflammation in the body. Chronic inflammation can contribute to joint pain and conditions like arthritis. Staying hydrated helps reduce the risk of inflammation.

5. Muscle Support: Hydration aids muscle function. Strong muscles provide better support to joints, reducing strain on them.

Herbal Teas for Joint Support

Certain herbal teas can provide additional joint support, complementing proper hydration:

1. Turmeric Tea: Turmeric contains curcumin, a compound known for its anti-inflammatory properties. Curcumin may help reduce joint pain and stiffness by targeting inflammation in the body. Turmeric tea is a popular choice for those seeking natural joint support.

2. Ginger Tea: Ginger has anti-inflammatory and analgesic properties that can provide relief from joint pain and swelling. Consuming ginger tea may help manage symptoms of osteoarthritis and other joint conditions.

3. Green Tea: Green tea contains antioxidants called catechins that possess anti-inflammatory effects. These antioxidants might help protect joint tissues and reduce the risk of cartilage degradation.

4. Nettle Leaf Tea: Nettle leaf is rich in vitamins and minerals that can contribute to joint health.

It has been traditionally used to alleviate symptoms of arthritis, as it may help reduce inflammation and improve joint function.

5. Chamomile Tea: Chamomile's anti-inflammatory and calming properties can indirectly support joint health by promoting relaxation and stress reduction. Chronic stress can worsen inflammatory conditions, so managing stress is essential for overall joint well-being.

6. Boswellia Tea: Boswellia, also known as Indian frankincense, contains compounds that have been studied for their potential anti-inflammatory effects. Boswellia tea might aid in reducing joint pain and improving mobility.

7. Rose Hip Tea: Rose hips are rich in vitamin C and antioxidants, which can support the immune system and joint health. The anti-inflammatory properties of rose hips may also contribute to their positive impact on joints.

It's important to note that while these herbal teas may offer potential benefits, individual responses can vary.

Herbal teas can be a complementary addition to a balanced diet, regular exercise, and proper medical care in supporting joint health.

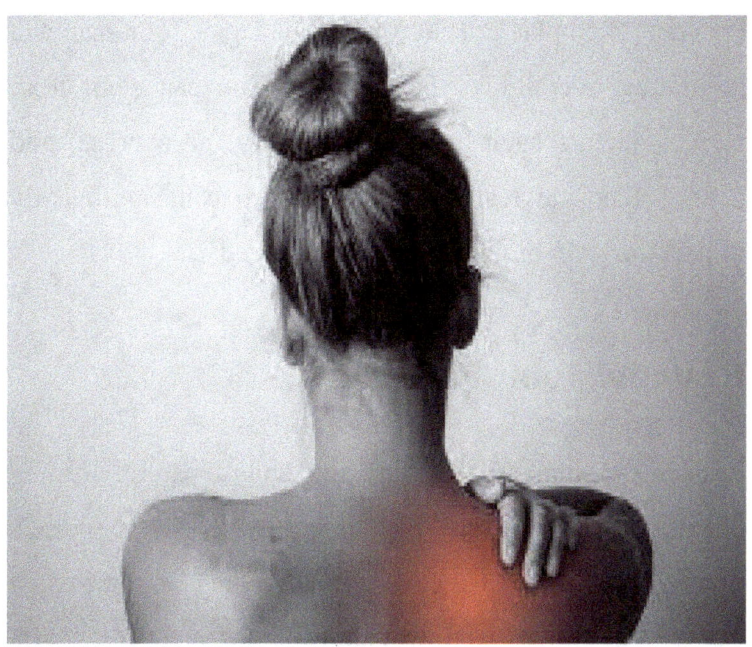

Chapter 12

Rest and Sleep

Rest and sleep play crucial roles in managing joint pain and promoting overall well-being. Joint pain can stem from various factors such as arthritis, injury, or overuse, and getting adequate rest and quality sleep can significantly impact the level of discomfort experienced.

Rest and Joint Pain

Rest is essential for allowing the body's natural healing processes to take place. When joints are overused or injured, they require time to recover. By avoiding activities that exacerbate the pain and providing the affected joints with adequate rest, you can help prevent further irritation and allow inflammation to subside.

However, prolonged immobilization can lead to stiffness and muscle weakening, so it's important to find a balance between rest and gentle movement.

Proper Sleep Positions

1. Choosing the right sleep positions can alleviate joint pain and provide a more restful sleep experience. For individuals with joint pain, certain sleep positions are more advantageous than others:

2. Back Sleeping: Sleeping on your back with a pillow under your knees can help maintain the natural curvature of your spine and alleviate pressure on your joints.

3. Side Sleeping: If you prefer sleeping on your side, place a pillow between your knees to keep your hips, pelvis, and spine properly aligned, reducing strain on your joints.

4. Avoid Stomach Sleeping: Sleeping on your stomach can lead to unnatural twisting of the neck and spine, potentially worsening joint pain.

Importance of Restful Sleep

Restful sleep is essential for everyone, but it holds particular significance for those dealing with joint pain:

1. Pain Reduction: During deep sleep stages, the body releases growth hormone, which aids in tissue repair. Quality sleep can help reduce inflammation and alleviate joint pain.

2. Tissue Repair: Sleep is a crucial time for the body to repair and rebuild tissues. For individuals with joint pain, this means that damaged joint tissues may have a better chance of healing during restful sleep.

3. Mood and Coping: Chronic joint pain can impact mood and mental well-being. Sleep plays a role in regulating mood, so obtaining sufficient sleep can help improve emotional resilience and coping with pain.

4. Energy Restoration: Quality sleep restores energy levels and enhances overall vitality. This can lead to better pain management during waking hours.

Rest and sleep are integral components of managing joint pain. By giving your body the time it needs to heal through proper rest and sleep, you can reduce inflammation, support tissue repair, and enhance your overall well-being.

Additionally, adopting suitable sleep positions can alleviate pressure on your joints, leading to a more comfortable and restful night's sleep.

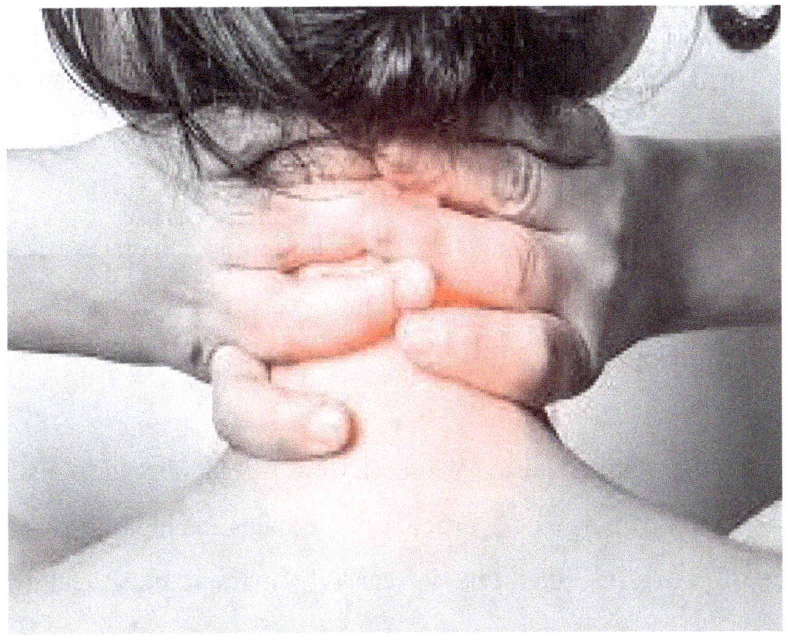

Chapter 13

Practical Tips for Daily Joint Care

Taking care of your joints is essential for maintaining overall mobility and reducing the risk of joint pain and discomfort. Here are some practical tips to help you with daily joint care:

1. Stay Active: Engage in regular low-impact exercises like walking, swimming, or cycling to keep your joints moving and maintain flexibility.

2. Maintain a Healthy Weight: Excess weight puts additional stress on your joints, particularly the knees and hips. The risk of joint issues might be decreased by maintaining a healthy weight.

3. Balanced Diet: Consume plenty of fruits and vegetables, whole grains, lean proteins, and healthy fats. Certain nutrients like omega-3 fatty acids can help reduce inflammation.

4. Stay Hydrated: Proper hydration supports the lubrication of joints, reducing friction and maintaining their function.

5. Proper Posture: Maintain good posture while sitting, standing, and lifting to reduce strain on your joints, especially your spine.

6. Joint-Friendly Supplements: Consult with a healthcare professional about supplements like glucosamine and chondroitin that can support joint health.

7. Wear Supportive Footwear: Choose shoes that provide proper arch support and cushioning to reduce impact on your knees and hips.

8. Avoid Repetitive Motions: Minimize activities that involve repetitive joint movements, as they can lead to overuse and strain.

9. Warm Up and Cool Down: Prior to exercise, warm up your joints with gentle stretches and movements. Afterward, cool down to help prevent stiffness.

Ergonomic Adjustments

Ergonomic adjustments involve optimizing your work or living environment to reduce strain on your joints and minimize discomfort. Consider the following tips:

1. Proper Seating and Posture: Use chairs with good lumbar support and cushioning. Maintain an upright posture, keeping your back straight and shoulders relaxed. Use footrests to support your feet if they don't reach the ground.

2. Ergonomic Workspace: Adjust the height and angle of your computer monitor to avoid straining your neck and eyes. Ensure your keyboard and mouse are at a comfortable height to prevent wrist and forearm strain.

3. Supportive Tools: Use ergonomic tools like keyboard and mouse pads with wrist support, as well as ergonomic office accessories to maintain neutral wrist, hand, and forearm positions.

4. Regular Breaks: Take short breaks to stretch and move around. This helps reduce joint stiffness and promotes blood circulation.

5. Avoiding Overexertion for Joint Pain:
Overexertion can exacerbate joint pain. Here's how to avoid it:

6. Listen to Your Body: Take note of your body's cues. If you experience pain, stop the activity and rest.

7. Moderation: Avoid excessive or sudden increases in physical activity. Gradually build up intensity and duration to give your joints time to adapt.

8. Proper Technique: Learn and use proper techniques for lifting, bending, and carrying objects. This keeps your joints from experiencing undue strain.

9. Weight Management: Maintaining a healthy weight reduces the load on your joints, especially those in the lower body.

Protecting Joints During Activities

Protecting your joints during activities helps prevent further damage and discomfort:

1. Warm-Up: Always perform a proper warm-up before engaging in physical activities. Gentle stretches and movements prepare your joints for more strenuous action.

2. Use Proper Equipment: When participating in sports or exercises, wear appropriate footwear and use necessary protective gear to minimize impact on your joints.

3. Range of Motion Exercises: Engage in regular exercises that promote joint flexibility and range of motion. Tai chi and yoga have advantages.

4. Low-Impact Activities: Choose activities that are easier on the joints, such as swimming, cycling, or walking, to maintain fitness without excessive strain.

Chapter 14

Seeking Professional Advice

Joint pain can significantly impact an individual's quality of life and daily activities. Seeking professional advice is crucial to properly diagnose the underlying cause and determine the most effective treatment options.

Joint pain can result from various factors, including injury, arthritis, inflammation, autoimmune disorders, or even an underlying medical condition.

Consulting a Doctor or Specialist

When experiencing joint pain, it's essential to consult a medical professional. A general practitioner can provide an initial evaluation, but if the pain is chronic or severe, consulting a specialist like a rheumatologist or an orthopedic surgeon might be necessary.

These specialists have expertise in diagnosing and treating joint-related issues and can recommend appropriate diagnostic tests, such as X-rays, MRI scans, or blood tests, to identify the root cause of the pain.

Integrating Natural Approaches with Medical Advice

While medical advice should always be the primary consideration for joint pain, integrating natural approaches can complement traditional treatments. Here are some ways to combine natural approaches with medical advice:

1. Healthy Lifestyle Choices: Maintaining a healthy weight through proper diet and regular exercise can alleviate joint stress. Low-impact exercises like swimming, yoga, and tai chi can improve flexibility and strength without straining the joints.

2. Dietary Changes: Some foods have anti-inflammatory properties that can help manage joint pain. Incorporating omega-3 fatty acids found in fish, flaxseeds, and walnuts, as

well as antioxidants from fruits and vegetables, can potentially reduce inflammation.

3. Supplements: Certain supplements like glucosamine and chondroitin sulfate have been studied for their potential benefits in managing joint pain. However, it's important to consult a healthcare professional before starting any new supplements.

4. Herbal Remedies: Turmeric and ginger are known for their anti-inflammatory properties and may provide relief for some individuals. Herbal remedies should be used cautiously and discussed with a doctor to avoid potential interactions with medications.

5. Physical Therapies: Modalities like heat and cold therapy, massage, and acupuncture can offer relief by promoting blood circulation, reducing muscle tension, and improving joint mobility.

6. Mind-Body Techniques: Practices such as meditation and deep breathing can help manage stress, which can indirectly

impact joint pain. Stress reduction techniques can be beneficial in overall pain management.

7. Hydration: Staying hydrated supports joint lubrication and overall bodily functions. Drinking an adequate amount of water can contribute to joint health.

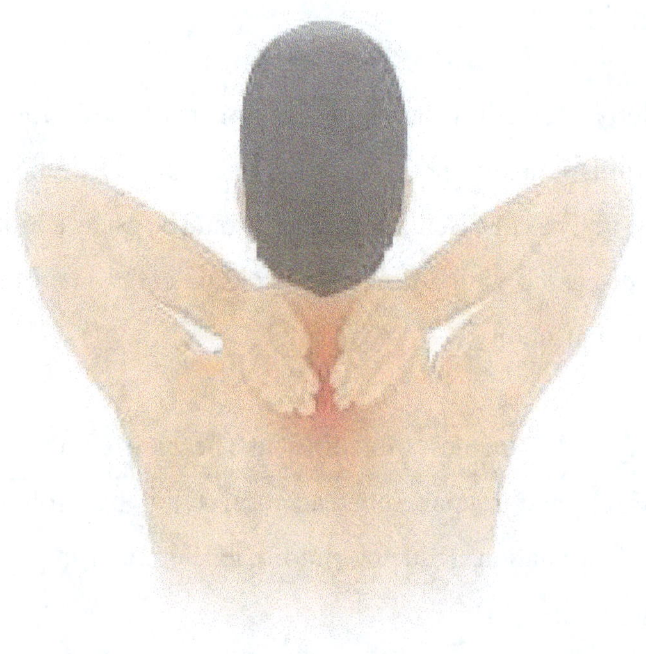

CHAPTER 15

Conclusion

Effective natural joint pain relief offers a promising approach to managing discomfort and improving overall quality of life.

The exploration of natural remedies, such as herbal supplements, dietary adjustments, and physical therapies, has shown encouraging results in alleviating joint pain.

These methods often provide a holistic approach that not only targets the symptoms but also addresses underlying causes.

The efficacy of natural joint pain relief can be attributed to their anti-inflammatory, analgesic, and nourishing properties.

Herbal supplements like turmeric, ginger, and boswellia have demonstrated their ability to reduce inflammation and provide pain relief. Incorporating a well-balanced diet rich in omega-3 fatty acids, antioxidants, and vitamins can further promote joint health and mitigate discomfort.

Physical therapies like yoga, tai chi, and low-impact exercises not only enhance joint flexibility but also aid in strengthening surrounding muscles.

This holistic approach fosters long-term joint health and minimizes the reliance on conventional medication.

However, it's important to note that individual responses may vary, and consultation with a healthcare professional is essential before adopting any natural remedies.

In severe cases, a combination of natural approaches and conventional medical interventions might yield the best results.

Ultimately, the pursuit of effective natural joint pain relief offers a complementary avenue for those seeking alternatives to traditional pharmaceutical solutions, promoting a more balanced and sustainable path to well-being.

Taking Charge of Your Joint Health

Maintaining optimal joint health is crucial for leading a healthy and active life. Joints play a pivotal role in our body, allowing movement and flexibility.

Whether you're a young adult or aging gracefully, taking proactive steps to care for your joints can significantly impact your overall well-being.

Here are some comprehensive tips and encouragement to help you take charge of your joint health:

1. Stay Active: Regular physical activity helps to keep your joints flexible and strong. Low-impact exercises like swimming, walking, and cycling can be especially beneficial without putting excess stress on the joints.

2. Maintain a Healthy Weight: Excess body weight places added strain on your joints, particularly on weight-bearing ones like knees and hips. By maintaining a healthy weight, you reduce the risk of joint-related problems.

3. Balanced Diet: A well-rounded diet rich in nutrients is essential for joint health. Omega-3 fatty acids found in fish, antioxidants from colorful fruits and vegetables, and vitamin D for bone health are particularly important.

4. Stay Hydrated: Proper hydration helps to keep your joints lubricated, reducing friction and discomfort. Water also supports the overall health of your connective tissues.

5. Protective Measures: When engaging in physical activities or sports, use proper protective gear such as knee pads, wrist guards, and helmets to prevent injuries that can affect your joints.

6. Proper Posture: Maintaining good posture helps distribute your body weight evenly and reduces strain on specific joints. This is especially important for your spine and neck.

7. Joint-Friendly Movements: Be mindful of your body mechanics while lifting heavy objects or performing repetitive tasks. Using proper techniques can prevent joint injuries.

8. Avoid Overuse: Repetitive motions can lead to overuse injuries. Incorporate variety into your activities to avoid placing excessive stress on the same joints repeatedly.

9. Warm-Up and Cool Down: Prior to exercise, warming up helps increase blood flow to your muscles and joints, reducing the risk of injury. Cooling down after exercise aids in the prevention of stiffness.

10. Strength Training: Building muscle strength around your joints provides added support. Focus on exercises that target the muscle groups surrounding specific joints.

11. Flexibility Exercises: Regular stretching routines enhance joint flexibility, allowing for a wider range of motion and reducing the risk of stiffness.

12. Listen to Your Body: Keep an eye out for any signs of joint discomfort or pain. Ignoring these red flags may result in more significant issues. Rest and get medical help if required.

13. Medical Check-ups: Regular check-ups with a healthcare professional, especially if you have a history of joint problems, can help identify issues early and provide appropriate guidance.

14. Medication and Supplements: Consult a healthcare provider before taking any joint health supplements or medications. Some supplements like glucosamine and chondroitin may provide benefits, but their effectiveness varies.

By incorporating these practices into your lifestyle, you can take proactive steps to safeguard your joint health, enhance your overall mobility, and enjoy an active life with fewer limitations. Always remember that personalized advice from healthcare professionals is essential for addressing individual needs and concerns.

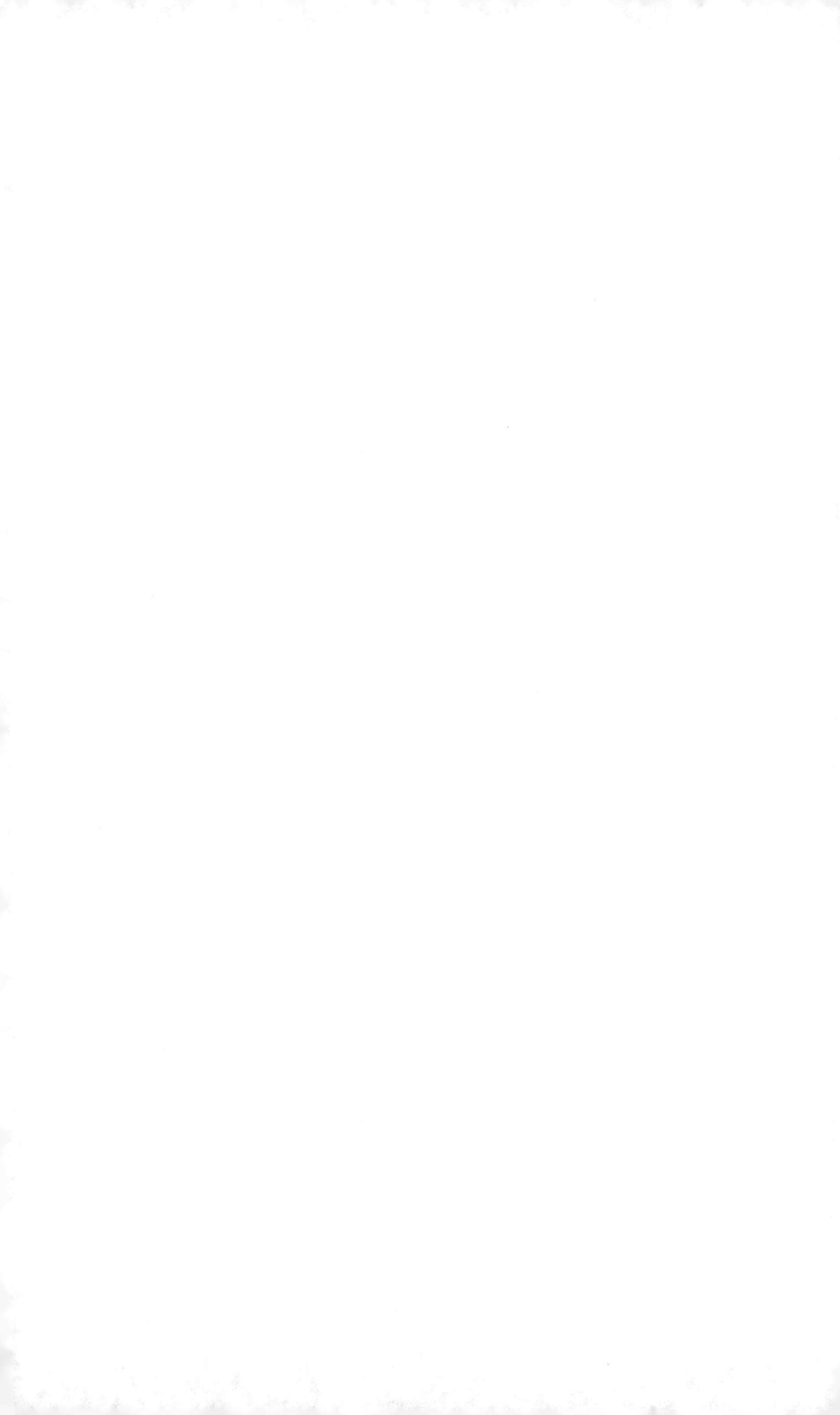